YOGASTROLOGY®
Yoga Meets Astrology

DIANE BOOTH GILLIAM, MA, E-RYT

Copyright © 2013 Diane Booth Gilliam All rights reserved

This book or parts thereof may not be reproduced without written permission. For further information and to contact the author, please visit yogastrology.com. With gratitude for your respect.

SECOND EDITION

ISBN: 1483996905
ISBN 13: 9781483996905

Photo Credits

Aries Marlize Joubert by Marlize Joubert; Taurus Marita Cooke of Yoga-Ninja.com by Libby Murfey; Gemini Kathryn Budig by Lululemon, and David Romanelli by Ken Goodman; Cancer Hemalayaa Behl by Trinity Wheeler, and Damiana Carpizo by Yogastrology.com; Leo Lacey Fedel by Lacey Fedel; Virgo Faith Hunter by Drew Xeron, and Sara LeVere by Victoria Ng; Libra Tiffany Cruikshank by BMAC Photography, and Elena Brower by Oshi Yuval; Scorpio Sadie Nardini by Sadie Nardini; Sagittarius Shakti Sunfire by Heather Van Buren; Capricorn Laurèn Rovira by Laurèn Rovira; Aquarius Leah Kim by David RE Photography; Pisces Dani Byrne McGuire by Rachael Jordan, Nancy Kate Williams Rau by Rick Cummings: main photo on front cover Karen Then by David Cook.

Yogastrology is a trademark registered with the United States Patent and Trademark Office. The exercise instructions and advice presented by Yogastrology are designed for people who are in good health and physically fit. They are not intended to substitute for medical counseling. The creators, producers, participants, Certified Yogastrology-Inspired and Certified Yogastrologers and distributors of Yogastrology disclaim any liability for loss or injury in connection with the exercises shown or the instruction and advice expressed.

WELCOME	V

HOW TO	IX

CHAPTER ONE	1

aries: HEAD

CHAPTER TWO	11

taurus: NECK & THROAT

CHAPTER THREE	19

gemini: SHOULDERS

CHAPTER FOUR	27

cancer: CHEST

CHAPTER FIVE	37

leo: SPINE

CHAPTER SIX	45

virgo: ABDOMEN

CHAPTER SEVEN — 55
libra: LOWER BACK

CHAPTER EIGHT — 63
scorpio: PELVIS

CHAPTER NINE — 71
sagittarius: HIPS

CHAPTER TEN — 79
capricorn: KNEES

CHAPTER ELEVEN — 87
aquarius: ANKLES

CHAPTER TWELVE — 95
pisces: FEET

NAMASTÉ — 103

WELCOME

I was a yoga teacher trekking around the colorful world of India. One morning, on the Full Moon, a friend whispered, "*Yagna* fire ceremony, in the village. Come."

Meandering through dusty streets, I found the address, ascended a steep staircase, and took a seat on the cool concrete floor. Soon I was engulfed in thick swirls of incense and loud, resonant Sanskrit chants. The traditional ceremonies ensued. My mind grew still.

The fire crackled.

Into that wide-open space drifted one thought: *There is some connection between yoga and astrology.*

Where that thought came from remains a mystery to this day. Believe me, over the years, I've tried to put that thought away and do something more...*ordinary*. Whatever it was, it had me by the tail.

Fast-forward a few years. Departed from India, settled back in the United States, my marriage was falling apart. I was trying to fit into a tiny rental, feeling raw and heartbroken when, unpacking a few boxes of possessions, yoga books, and old magazines about natural health, suddenly a publication fell open on the floor, revealing a chart. Hidden deep in the secrets of natural healing, an elegant tradition correlated areas of the human body with zodiac signs.

Spellbound, I couldn't take my eyes off that chart. I toted it to the computer, sat down, and started typing, aligning traditional body–zodiac correlations with yoga. The words flowed together seamlessly.

Yogastrology was born.

This book is your personal guide to Yogastrology for your zodiac sign and for every zodiac sign. Use it every month: Sync your yoga practice with the energies of the current month and embody new strength and fresh vitality all year.

These twelve chapters contain the month-to-month Yogastrology protocol:

- Astrological signs, natural elements, ruling planets
- Traditional body–zodiac correlations, asana suggestions, yogic explorations
- Journaling exercises, healing mantras, empowering affirmations

One of my favorite new features in this edition of the book is the Yogastrology Community, composed of A-list yogis David Romanelli,

Elena Brower, Faith Hunter, Hemalayaa Behl, Kathryn Budig, Leah Kim, Sadie Nardini, Shakti Sunfire, Tiffany Cruikshank, and more.

The yogis, who appear with their zodiac signs, share insights and flesh out the yoga-meets-astrology connection. They help us "get" Yogastrology.

To learn more, visit Yogastrology.com Community webpage and Training webpage, where you will meet our students and graduates of our training programs, and hear what exciting things they're up to in their yoga classes and workshops.

I offer my gratitude to the yogis in the Yogastrology Community, and to you, the reader. I bow to that magical, wide-open space within us where miracles happen.

Namasté,

Diane Booth Gilliam, MA, E-RYT

traditional zodiac : BODY correlations

aries : HEAD

taurus : NECK

gemini : SHOULDERS

cancer : CHEST

leo : SPINE

virgo : ABDOMEN

libra : LOW BACK

scorpio : PELVIS

sagittarius : HIPS

capricorn : KNEES

aquarius : ANKLES

pisces : FEET

HOW TO

Here are four ways to use Yogastrology.

1. Yogastrology for your zodiac (Sun) sign.

Hatha yoga means Sun (ha) and Moon (tha) in Sanskrit.

Yogastrology is a compelling new path. Use it to explore astrology, expand your hatha yoga practice, and embrace radical self-acceptance. Use it for stellar wellness.

Check out the chapter for your sign.

2. Yogastrology for the current zodiac (Sun) sign.

Yogastrology is your guide throughout the year.

Every month, the Sun moves (ingresses) into a different zodiac sign. For example, the sign of Aries begins March 21 and ends April 19.

When we embody the qualities of the current month's zodiac sign *at the right time, during the month when the sign is at its most succulent ripeness,* we embrace our own multi-dimensionality and become the rich, luscious, vibrant human beings we are meant to be. Yogastrology is your guide to embody the strengths of the current sign.

3. Yogastrology attuned with the rhythms of the Moon.

Yogastrology practices for the monthly New Moon and Full Moon are rich and varied. Every lunation has its own incomparable power.

Yogastrology training guides you to align, in your own unique way, with the power that is inherent in the phases of the Moon. Visit us at Yogastrology.com to learn more.

4. Yogastrology's fresh seasonal practices.

Yogastrology promotes optimal well-being in sync with the four seasons, solstices, equinoxes, and the four elements of astrology–fire, earth, air, and water. Sense the seething passion of fire. Touch the noble earth. Breathe fresh mountain air. Bathe in deep healing waters.

Immerse yourself in the transformative power of Yogastrology. Unleash your highest potential.

Notes

The energy of astrological events builds and then peaks at one exact moment in time. The effects linger for several hours, days, or longer.

Yogastrology works with both Western astrology and Vedic astrology. The foundation of Yogastrology is an ancient tradition of body–zodiac correlations (for example, Aries = head) and these correlations are very similar in both Western and Vedic astrology. In this book, Yogastrology uses Western astrological dates because most people are familiar with the Western astrology zodiac.

The dates in the book are approximate. Slight variations in the dates may occur year to year, and according to geographical locations and time zones.

1 aries: HEAD

Sun in Aries: March 21 to April 19

Welcome to Aries Yogastrology. This chapter invites you to honor your inner fire, and relax. Restful relaxation helps you rejuvenate and get ahead.

1.1 Element, Overview, Ruling Planet: Mars
1.2 Traditional Body–Zodiac Correlation: Head
1.3 Wellness: Asanas
1.4 Exploration: Ganesha, the Remover of Obstacles
1.5 Journaling: What makes you hot?
1.6 Community: Marlize Joubert, Aries
1.7 Affirmation: I grant myself the right to relax.

Have you ever had answers come when you're doing yoga? Suddenly you "get" it–a problem is solved or you see which way to go. When you relax and let tension melt away, higher wisdom comes through.

Go ahead, relax...and get *ahead*.

1.1 Aries Element, Overview, Ruling Planet

The zodiac is divided into four elements–fire, earth, air, and water; each element correlates with three zodiac signs.

Aries is the first of three fire signs (Aries, Leo, Sagittarius).

It is the very first sign in the zodiac.

First is not an easy place to be. It takes courage, stamina, and moxie to go ahead of the pack. When it's your turn to go first, be sure that your personal trailblazing has a clear direction, and you have set an intention or goal.

Be sure you know when to charge ahead (Aries's specialty), as well as when it's time to relax and let things percolate for a while (let *Shavasana* help with the latter).

Aries's symbol, the ram, suggests the appropriate energy needed to ramrod into new terrain. Aries packs a fiery punch, for sure. This zodiac sign represents energy, desire, and passion.

Ruling planet: Mars

By Dana Gerhardt | Used by permission of the author

Mars likes action. Notwithstanding the media's lust for violence, most of us lead relatively safe and quiet lives. This puts many a Mars warrior behind a desk, staring at a computer, attending business meetings, shopping, doing the laundry, maybe fantasizing on porn sites, or watching a privileged few athletes parade their Mars on TV.

But Mars doesn't go happily into domesticated bliss, a fact even Madison Avenue has noticed. Witness the recent Burger King commercial converting the feminist anthem "I am woman" into a resounding *manthem*, declaring "I am man. I've had enough of chick food. I need to wrap my sturdy hands around a burger!"

Mars is not delicate. In the Star Trek universe, he would have been a Klingon. He's bursting with raw physical vitality. He's fiery and impulsive, also competitive and selfish. He's the anger we don't like to admit, the illicit passion we work to transcend. He's also powerful, independent, and courageous. With the force of Mars we can climb mountains, wage ambitious campaigns, protect the defenseless, stand for what we believe.

But listen to conversations around the water cooler and you'll find more people criticize Mars expressions than cheer them on. "Allen is so competitive." "Did you hear the mean remark Emily said?" Mars is what other people have that gives us trouble. If we bring our own Mars into an astrology reading, we often do it indirectly, complaining how we're tired all the time, or not "getting any," or that we hate what we do.

Of course the real problem may be that our assertive lusty Mars is idling....

1.2 Traditional Body–Zodiac Correlation

Aries: Head

Also: Face, brain, blood, muscular action, and adrenal glands

1.3 Wellness: Asanas

The cusp of Aries, on or around March 21, signifies balance. This is the Spring Equinox in the northern hemisphere, Autumnal Equinox in the southern hemisphere.

The word "equinox" means equal night. Day and night are of equal length–in balance.

Align with Equinox energy by practicing balance poses, such as *Vrksasana,* tree pose.

All yoga is good. For Aries, practice any asana (at any level, beginner to advanced, whatever is appropriate for you) while maintaining focus on the head. You might try the following practices:

Uttanasana, standing forward bend

Janu Sirsasana, head-to-knee pose

Salamba Sirsasana, supported headstand

Kapalabhati Pranayama, skull shining breath

Pincha Mayurasana, feathered peacock pose

Prasarita Padottanasana, wide-legged forward bend

Virabhadrasana, warrior pose (any variation) honoring the warrior planet, Mars

Featured Asana: *Shavasana,* sponge or corpse pose

Shavasana is a beautiful practice for contending with the busyness of the mind that plagues us human beings. I have spent vast amounts of time and energy analyzing this question: Why can't we just relax? Finally, I considered this possibility.

Let's give our personal layers of muck (and we all have muck) the respect it deserves. And then be done with it. Let the muck be seen, heard, and acknowledged, without poring over it endlessly. Get it out. Honor it. And then be willing to let it go.

Our minds change, our thoughts change. Much of what fills our heads is so fleeting, if we are willing to let it go. Thoughts are like clouds in the sky. Watch them come, watch them go. We can always return to center, a place of inner serenity and balance.

If you experience distractions when practicing Shavasana, try calling on Ganesha. Ask this ancient symbol of benevolent grace to help remove obstacles that stand in the way of your relaxation and your full experience of Shavasana.

1.4 Exploration

Ganesha is the elephant-headed one. His image is placed over doorways in India, as Ganesha honors the importance of beginnings and bestows blessings on each new endeavor. Marriage, a new business, any new undertaking–these are Ganesha's domain.

Realize how every obstacle we encounter is placed in our lives to help us learn and grow in exactly the way we need to.

Call on Ganesha. Ask for his help in removing obstacles blocking your way. He is known for his benevolence. One of his songs, the "Ganesha Gayatri Mantra," offers protection:

Om Ekadantaya Vidmahe

Vakkratundaya Dheemahi

Tanno Danti Prachodayat

We devote our thoughts to the one-tusked lord.

We meditate upon him who has a curved trunk.

May the tusked one guide us on the right path.

1.5 Journaling

Ask yourself, "What makes me hot?" "Where is my lusty, aggressive, angry, passionate, assertive Mars fire?"

Get started exploring this. You might set a timer for twenty minutes, more or less, to explore this. Recall, imagine, dance, sing, write, draw, scribble, color. You name it.

And please note: You don't have to color inside the lines. You can get messy; you don't have to act nice.

Go ahead. Grab a pen and paper. Explore your Mars–Aries fire. Do whatever you want to do to offer tribute to Mars.

ZZZ the timer's buzzer goes off. Did you get it all out? If not, keep going. "Get it out of your system," as my mother would say.

If you are reading this book with others, then pair off and share what you discovered about your inner Aries energy and your Mars fire.

Use the journaling exercises. Combined with the practices of yoga, they are great for freeing up energy, moving forward, and charging ahead (Aries's specialty).

1.6 Community

Marlize Joubert, Aries

It has taken me a long time to slow down. When I first started practicing yoga, I left early! I didn't understand the whole concept of Shavasana.

Now, after years of practice, I have slowed down enough that Shavasana has become my favorite pose. It drops me deeper into myself each time I practice, and as I begin to meet myself on a deeper level, I notice how amazing it feels.

And so I began to find Shavasana in everything I do: standing in the grocery line or watching an elderly couple walk hand-in-hand.

Relaxation came when I was ready to appreciate it. As we grow, we discover, we heal, we learn, we remember what is important in life.

1.7 Affirmation

I grant myself the right to relax.

All the hemispheres in heaven
Are sitting around a Fire
Chatting
While stitching themselves together
Into the Great Circle inside of You.
-Hafiz

1 ARIES: HEAD | 9

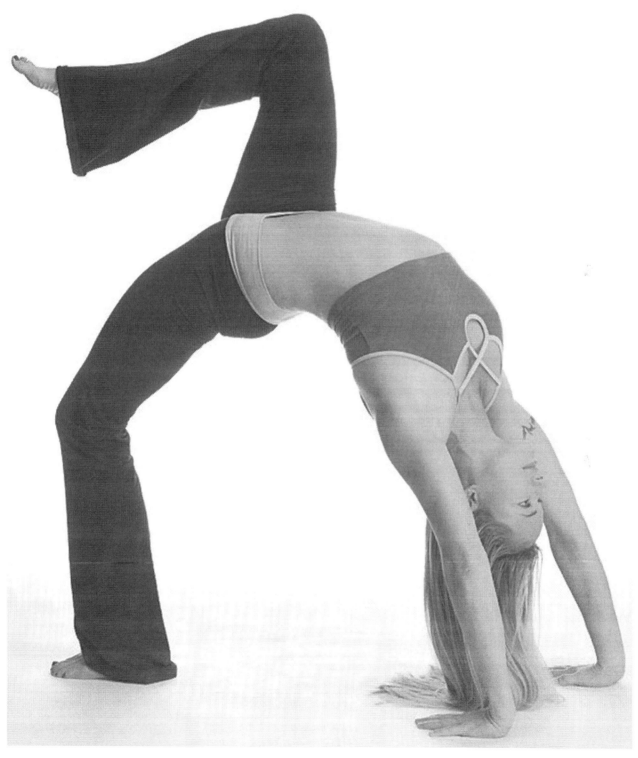

Marlize Joubert

2 taurus: NECK & THROAT

Sun in Taurus: April 20 to May 20

Welcome to Taurus Yogastrology. This chapter leads you to explore what true abundance means to you.

2.1 Element, Overview, Ruling Planet: Venus
2.2 Traditional Body–Zodiac Correlation: Neck & Throat
2.3 Wellness: Asanas
2.4 Exploration: OM and the Fifth Chakra
2.5 Journaling: What makes life rich?
2.6 Community: Marita Cooke, Taurus
2.7 Affirmation: I live in abundance.

Hello soothing neck stretches, goodbye pain in the neck.

You're sure to find much more in this chapter to make life rich, abundant, and buzzing with the resonance of OM.

2.1 Taurus Element, Overview, Ruling Planet

Taurus is the first of three earth signs (Taurus, Virgo, Capricorn). This sign imparts a feeling of calm and persistence, and it's easy to see the determination; the influence of Taurus tends to make a person move slowly and deliberately.

Taurus is warmhearted, stable, reliable, and security loving. The other side of his nature might be jealousy or possessiveness.

Occasionally, Taurus can be inflexible. And once in a great while, he may be capable of acting like a pain in the neck.

The symbol for Taurus, the bull, is known for its strength, stamina, and stability. The bull is a representation of wealth and abundance. A strong Taurus influence makes us peaceful, placid, and patient.

Ruling planet: Venus

Astrologer Dana Gerhardt is one of my favorite authors when it comes to the planets. So, naturally I was intrigued when she interviewed a few hundred people as part of a recent study she conducted. Her subject: Venus.

The results are in, and I love how Gerhardt presents the love goddess planet. Rather than making Venus take a hot shower, balance her checkbook, and blow-dry her hair before we can meet her, we see Venus after she's had a long day or some nasty scene from her too-busy life.

Now, of course, the Goddess of Love is still totally gorgeous. And she's sweaty, passionate, and ripe, too. Finally, she has Venusian multidimensionality, just like you and I and the rest of the real-life human goddesses do. Gerhardt paints a picture that is racy and vulnerable, raucous and vivacious. And I, for one, am happy to hear the truth about this glorious goddess of desire, love, and money.

By Dana Gerhardt | Used by permission of the author

> The goddess who craves pleasure and passion loves variety and intensity, which can be exhilarating.
>
> It's also disruptive, inspiring choices that shame or humiliate us, sending us to lovers who aren't good for us, into orgies of consumption we later regret, stimulating jealousy, inadequacy, and fear of loss.
>
> As an archetype, Venus maps our route to happiness. But she refuses to take only safe, well-lit roads. By her very nature, she keeps turning us into the dark.

2.2 Traditional Body–Zodiac Correlation

Taurus: Neck and throat

Also: Cervical spine and thyroid gland

2.3 Wellness: Asanas

The Sanskrit name for the fifth chakra (subtle-body energy center), located in the neck and throat, is *Vishuddha*, which means purity.

Every chakra is associated with a color. The fifth chakra is a brilliant blue, like the color of the peacock's long, shiny neck. It is said that the peacock is fully aware of his own beauty, which makes this exquisite creature even more confident and regal in stature.

All yoga is good. For Taurus, practice any asana (at any level, beginner to advanced, whatever is appropriate for you) while maintaining focus on the neck and throat. You might try the following practices:

Bitilasana, cow pose

Marjaryasana, cat pose

Trikonasana, triangle pose

Mayurasana, peacock pose

Viparita Karani, legs-up-the-wall pose

Setu Bandha Sarvangasana, bridge pose

Ardha Matsyendrasana, half lord of the fishes pose

Featured Asana: *Halasana*, plow pose

When you practice Halasana, be particularly mindful of your throat and the presence of the fifth chakra.

Deficient energy in the fifth chakra can cause neck stiffness or pain, fear of speaking, and other neck and throat ailments.

Excessive energy in the fifth chakra can cause hearing problems, reluctance to listen, and excessive talking.

Balance energy in the fifth chakra through asana practice and mantra repetition.

2.4 Exploration

Repetition of the mantra OM can transform one's speech, body, and mind into a beautiful state of exaltation.

The fifth chakra is purified by repetition of OM. As the fifth chakra becomes increasingly purer, we begin to understand our own inner truth. And we are able to speak our truth much more easily.

Sacred singing, speaking, reading aloud, and chanting enhance the well-being and the purification of this special chakra.

The entire body, down to the cellular level, is affected by the vibration of the voice, especially when you are repeating the sacred syllable OM.

2.5 Journaling

Ask yourself, "What makes life rich?"

What comes to your mind and body first? What is your first reaction, your initial response to the question, "What makes life rich?"

Take the opportunity to explore that now, and write about it. Or dance and sing your richness, if you want.

2.6 Community

Marita Cooke, Taurus

> Neck health is very personal to me.
>
> In 2005, I was in the perfect storm of a car accident, and it is a miracle that I survived. My neck suffered intense pain. It was immobilizing.
>
> My yoga practice has been a critical part of the journey and the reinvention of myself on many levels.
>
> Through the gift of yoga, my neck has become a source of strength and a testament to the power of this divine practice.

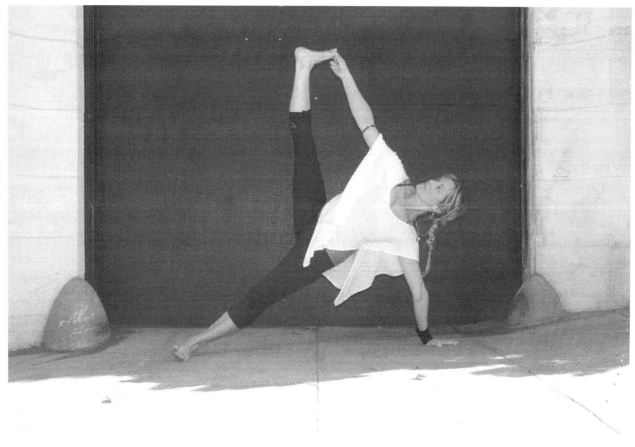

Marita Cooke

2.7 Affirmation

I live in abundance.

We have no art. We simply do everything as beautifully as we can.
-Balinese saying

3 gemini: SHOULDERS

Sun in Gemini: May 21 to June 21

Welcome to Gemini Yogastrology. This chapter inspires you to let burdens roll off your shoulders and breathe easily.

3.1 Element, Overview, Ruling Planet: Mercury
3.2 Traditional Body–Zodiac Correlation: Shoulders
3.3 Wellness: Asanas
3.4 Exploration: Pranayama
3.5 Journaling: How flexible am I?
3.6 Community: Kathryn Budig, Gemini; and David Romanelli, Gemini
3.7 Affirmation: I allow burdens to slide off my shoulders.

Gemini, the Twins, can be so two-sided, so over stuffed with information. Sounds like life, doesn't it? Information overload!

I chose only the juiciest tidbits to share with you in this chapter so you can stretch out, relax, and enjoy Gemini.

3.1 Gemini Element, Overview, Ruling Planet

Gemini is the first of three air signs (Gemini, Libra, Aquarius).

Gemini loves to think and talk, talk, talk. Not just idle chatter, either. Gemini goes for incessant exploration–people, places, and things–the more information the better. And Gemini loves to share what he's learned.

Gemini's influence also can make a person flighty and flirtatious. Enjoy the show because bright, funny Gemini is (or wants to be) the life of the party. He is hyperactive in the rationalization department too, so don't expect a straight answer. Entertaining diatribes, yes. Plenty of fun facts, too. Can Gemini be boring? Never.

The brightest stars in the Gemini constellation are named Castor and Pollux, which are also the names of mythological twins who are associated in art and literature with horses, symbolizing movement.

Ruling planet: Mercury

Mercury is the fastest-moving planet in the entire solar system. It's difficult to study because of its close proximity to the Sun, but we know that Mercury's days are hotter than a furnace, and the nights are cooler than a freezer.

Mercury is another name for the chemical element known as quicksilver. It's also the Latin name for the Greek god Hermes and the root of the word "merchandise," implying a connection between Mercury and trade, travel, and commercial affairs.

Qualities bestowed by chatty Mercury, astrologically speaking, include rapid change; the influence of Mercury imparts a keen interest in learning new things. Mercury is a shape-shifter, a trickster introducing a mosaic of moods, attitudes, and thoughts.

Mercury indicates intellectual style and daily communication, speech, and writing; he may lack depth and wisdom, but offers an entertaining, quick wit, with plenty of interesting news to share. Mercury is the fleet-footed winged messenger of the gods.

3.2 Traditional Body–Zodiac Correlation

Gemini: Shoulders

Also: Lungs, arms, hands, and fingers

3.3 Wellness: Asanas

No wonder we talk about shouldering responsibility. The muscles and joints of the shoulders must be flexible enough to accommodate the extraordinarily wide range of motion required by the arms and hands. Shoulders can:

- Abduct
- Adduct
- Rotate
- Rise in front of the torso
- Rise behind the torso
- Move through the full 360° plane

This tremendous range of motion makes the shoulder the most mobile joint in the human body. And it's more prone to dislocation and injury than any other joint.

Shoulders have to be flexible, but they also must be strong enough to support upper-body activities, such as pushing, pulling, and lifting. Do yoga to improve flexibility and strength.

All yoga is good. For Gemini, practice any asana (at any level, beginner to advanced, whatever is appropriate for you) while maintaining focus on the shoulders. You might try the following practices:

Tittibhasana, firefly pose

Dhanurasana, bow pose

Garudhasana, eagle pose

Bhujangasana, cobra pose

Gomukhasana, cow face pose

Utthita Parsvakonasana, extended side angle pose

Adho Mukha Svanasana, downward-facing dog pose

Featured Asana: *Parivritta Balasana,* thread-the-needle pose

In Parivritta Balasana, *ida* and *pingala* (two central nadis, or energy channels, in the subtle body) are crossed. When these two nadis cross one another, a wonderful sense of ease happens.

The tendency to slip into information overload, and the erratic changes introduced by the influence of planetary ruler Mercury, make this sense of ease especially welcome.

3.4 Exploration

It is the rare yoga student who is drawn immediately to *pranayama* (various breathing techniques to extend the *prana*–the body's rhythmic internal energy). Most people go to yoga class wanting to learn poses, sculpt and tone their bodies, maybe relax a little. Some go to meet beautiful people. I'm all for that. When I came to yoga, I entered through the door marked "Physical Body." Many years passed before the more subtle aspects of yoga, such as conscious breathing, popped up for me. The notion of using prana seemed like a distraction from my asana practice. Years after my first class, I began to understand that traditionally, pranayama was the core of hatha yoga practice. I'm a believer now. Experiencing the benefits of pranayama did it for me.

Pranayama is as simple as guiding your breath. The benefits of pranayama are profound, calming, and especially good for lungs or frazzled nerves.

3.5 Journaling

Ask yourself, "How flexible am I?"

- In my body?
- In my life?

How we are in our bodies is a mirror for how we are in our lives.

3.6 Community

Kathryn Budig, Gemini

> I've struggled with shoulder injuries throughout my yoga career. I believe they've all come from over-applying myself and not allowing the proper amount of rest to counteract my drive.
>
> It's a reminder to stay balanced with ambition and domestic bliss.
>
> I was actually supposed to be an identical twin, but she didn't make it through the pregnancy. Being a Gemini, I feel like she's my guardian angel, constantly steering me towards balance and wise choices. And I miss her.

3 GEMINI: SHOULDERS | 25

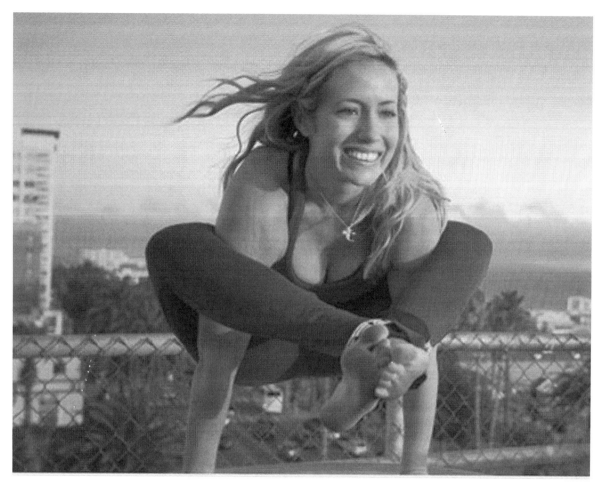

Kathryn Budig

David Romanelli, Gemini

> I could never wrap my head around astrology. Then one of my friends summed it up. He said, "You can travel with a map, or no map. Why not have a map?"
>
> My astrologer says I'm a mega-Gemini. I have all the strengths and weaknesses of the sign, magnified. It's so true. I have to talk about everything, anything. Some would say too much. But if you like to talk things through, I can do it for hours.

Trusting the journey has been difficult for me, and I think that's why I turned to yoga. You teach what you are learning—which makes it super-authentic.

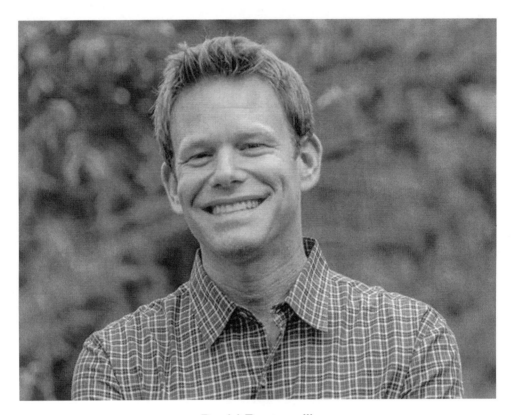

David Romanelli

3.7 Affirmation

I allow burdens to slide off my shoulders.

The Self-ing game is what Infinity does for fun.
-Jean Houston

4 cancer: CHEST

Sun in Cancer: June 22 to July 22

Welcome to Cancer Yogastrology. This chapter invites you to meet the Moon Goddess and avail yourself of her special gifts.

4.1 Element, Overview, Ruling Planet: the Moon
4.2 Traditional Body–Zodiac Correlation: Chest
4.3 Wellness: Asanas
4.4 Exploration: The Moon Goddess
4.5 Journaling: What is your connection with moonlight?
4.6 Community: Hemalayaa Behl, Cancer; and Damiana Carpizo, Cancer
4.7 Affirmation: I have a strong, protected, happy heart.

Cycles of the Moon present us with new opportunities every month. At the New Moon, meditate on new beginnings and set intentions. At the Full Moon, express fully and savor the fruits of your actions.

4.1 Cancer Element, Overview, Ruling Planet

Cancer marks the Solstice: Summer Solstice in the northern hemisphere, and Winter Solstice in the southern hemisphere.

Cancer is the first of three water signs (Cancer, Scorpio, Pisces). Water signs denote an emotional nature and, like Cancer's symbol the crab, an affinity for the sea.

This sign's characteristics are like those of a crab, a hard, protective shell on the outside, with soft and tender insides. Cancer represents the powerful, fertile female force of nature: Womanhood. Motherhood. Nourishment. Its shadow side includes devouring and grasping, holding tight with those crab claws that will not let go.

Cancer represents stereotypical femininity: attractive and passive; receptive; and reflective like the Moon, which rules Cancer.

Ruling planet: the Moon

While not technically a ruling "planet," the Moon is nevertheless a powerfully mysterious light that illuminates the dark night.

No one is immune to the magic of the Moon muse—not even the oceans. She entices us to swim in deep mystery and dance with high tides.

Representing primordial femininity, and reflecting the light of the Sun, the Moon and its regular cycles have been honored by countless people throughout time.

In astrology, your Moon sign holds high rank; it's one of the top three signs in terms of importance. While the Sun sign illuminates one's identity and purpose and the Rising sign comes up first to greet the world, the Moon sign shines on whatever the heart calls home: our habits and comfort zones; our emotional needs and responses. It also illuminates our neediness and how we project that neediness on others, especially our partners (and our mothers).

The Moon remembers. Somewhere under the light of the Moon lies a deep memory of infant-you, crying out in your crib, wailing in want of a nurturing stroke or a warm breast or bottle.

Your Moon remembers whether your needs were met and by whom. The Moon's placement and astrological aspects describe your interpretation of how you were mothered, comforted, and coddled, or smothered or manipulated.

Psychologists and astrologers usually claim that our memories dictate current and future relationships, and old habits die hard. Our habits drive our life choices in certain directions. We negotiate romantic relationships in terms of our astrological Moon. And eventually, if the Moon Goddess is willing, we come home to nest in the soft glow of moonlight, in the arms of a perfect partner.

4.2 Traditional Body–Zodiac Correlation

Cancer: Chest

Also: Womb and breasts–the body's feminine vessels that provide nurturance

4.3 Wellness: Asanas

The practices of yoga detoxify and calm the body and mind. Each one of the yogic practices, in its own way, purifies and uplifts us.

Scriptural study–of Patanjali's *Yoga Sutras*, the various Gitas, and more–clears the mind.

Chanting and mantra repetition clear the subtle body and the emotional body.

Hatha yoga clears the physical body.

Our memories are stored within our bodies. Everyone has had many experiences, and some were blissful. Some were not. Every memory is stored in the body.

Yoga goes deep, like a well, and taps into the Source that is flowing like a river, beneath the surface of life. The practices of yoga help us, on every level, to be calm and centered, strong and clear.

All yoga is good. For Cancer, practice any asana (at any level, beginner to advanced, whatever is appropriate for you) while maintaining focus on the chest. You might try the following practices:

Dhanurasana, bow pose

Bhujangasana, cobra pose

Purvottanasana, upward plank pose

Ardha Chandrasana, half moon pose

Natarajasana, lord of the dance pose

Setu Bandha Sarvangasana, bridge pose

Chandra Bhedana Pranayama, single nostril breath (Moon Piercing)

Featured Asana: *Chandra Namaskar,* Salutation to the Moon

According to hatha yoga, solar and lunar forces also reside within us. While solar energy is warm, active, and outwardly oriented, lunar energy is cool, receptive, and inwardly focused.

Chandra Namaskar is a meditative sequence that honors the Moon, lunar force, and nurturing feminine energy.

4.4 Exploration

Known as Diana to the Romans (also sometimes identified as Selene or Hecate), the Moon Goddess, Artemis, is one of the principal goddesses of Greek mythology. She is the protector of all women, and it is said that she does not consort with, nor bow to, the rule of any man.

She is the Huntress Goddess, the chief hunter of all gods and goddesses.

Though she is a huntress, she abhors violence and swiftly doles out punishment to offenders, especially those who threaten or harass women. The Goddess of the Hunt is known to frolic with, and occasionally slay, wild animals.

The mysteries of nature reveal themselves to her, and she, in turn reveals the depths of nature to those who seek her out, to those who seek to rest and regain strength in natural places.

Diana, or Artemis, is the protector of nature, of the wilderness, and of womankind.

4.5 Journaling

Ask yourself, "What is my connection with moonlight?"

The Goddess of the Moon offers protection, and those who have this protection are very fortunate.

Have you felt her protection? Have you sensed the Moon sharing secrets with you?

Let's offer gratitude. Write a poem or a love letter to the Moon Goddess to express your gratitude.

May you know how worthy you are and ask for a boon from the Moon Goddess. Seek her guidance; request special protection for yourself or for someone you love.

4.6   Community

Hemalayaa Behl, Cancer

> I am moody, and I love my home. Also I've been told I'm a very loving person.
>
> I feel a lot of sensitivity in my chest area, and I tend to be centered in my heart, physically and emotionally.
>
> Being a sensual Cancer, I guide yoga practice with a lot of sounds that are on the side of "yogasmic." It gets crazy in that yoga space!
>
> Try making sounds beyond the "sigh" sound in your practice, and see what happens.

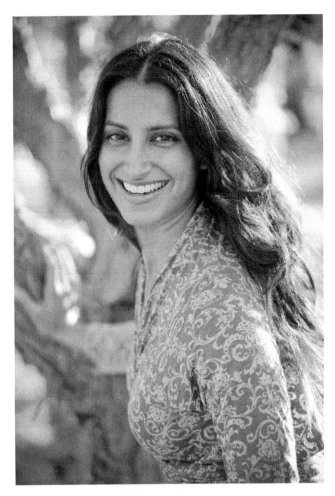

Hemalayaa Behl

Damiana Carpizo, Cancer

Openheartedness is a life theme for me. It is the place from which I seek to live.

The chest is the place in the body that is about openheartedness, nurturing, and receiving love. I think I am very good at all of these.

I'm a typical Cancer. Sensitive. Nurturing. Foodie. Outwardly protective of a luscious and delightful inside. And the best part is that I have a choice, every moment, about how to live.

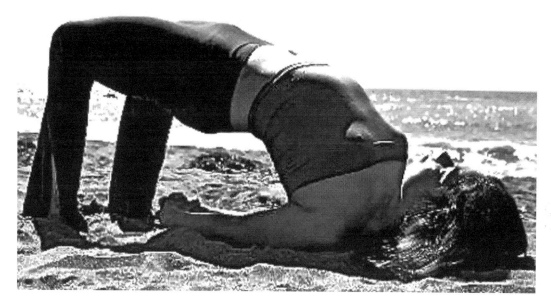

Damiana Carpizo

4.7 Affirmation

I have a strong, protected, happy heart.

> If you want to know the Truth, I can so clearly see that God has made love with you. And the whole universe is germinating inside your belly. And wonderful words, such enlightening words will take birth from you and be cradled against thousands of hearts.
> -Hafiz

5 leo: SPINE

Sun in Leo: July 23 to August 22

Welcome to Leo Yogastrology. This chapter leads you to find your courage and revel in it.

5.1 Element, Overview, Ruling Planet: the Sun
5.2 Traditional Body–Zodiac Correlation: Spine
5.3 Wellness: Asanas
5.4 Exploration: Surya, the Most Visible Form of Divinity
5.5 Journaling: What is in the book of your life?
5.6 Community: Lacey Fedel, Leo
5.7 Affirmation: I respect my courage.

Use this chapter as a guide to honor your spine—the backbone of your body and the backbone of your life. Respect your very own courageous self.

5.1 Leo Element, Overview, Ruling Planet

Leo is a bold and beautiful zodiac sign. While not technically a ruling "planet," the Sun rules this sign, and the astrological element for Leo is fire.

Qualities of Leo include confidence, sincerity, and enthusiasm. Leo is outgoing and likable; he also tends to be self-indulgent and luxury loving.

One of the most dynamic qualities of Leo is a flair for the dramatic. Leo is flashy and shiny like his ruler, the Sun.

He likes to receive praise, too—he might pout, or growl, if he doesn't receive it.

The constellation Leo signifies bravery and magnificence, such as we find displayed in the regal symbol for Leo, the lion.

At times, a Leo may sport an inborn feeling of superiority, and he might suffer from self-centeredness. But he won't suffer for long. Leo's natural authoritarian streak has him back in the saddle in no time. Proud, dignified, bright, and courageous—Leo is the shining star of the zodiac.

Ruling planet: the Sun

The Sun illuminates everything in its path. It is the source of life in our solar system, and in astrology, your personal Sun says a lot about your unique source of strength. To put it another way, the astrological Sun is one of the primary indicators of identity and purpose in life, as well as how to go about achieving that purpose.

Almost everybody knows his or her zodiac Sun sign. If you are a Leo, that means the Sun was located (from our vantage point here on earth) in the constellation Leo at the moment of your birth.

Many factors, especially Sun, Moon, and Rising signs, can be taken into consideration in a personal astrology chart reading; that's why not all people born under one Sun sign are alike.

Then again, every month *we are all one.* We are united under the Sun (and the zodiac Sun sign of the month).

During each monthly sign—the month of Leo, for example—Yogastrology guides people of every sign to tap into the power and strength of the current sign; in this case, it's all about Leonine energy.

That is the strength of Yogastrology, and it's one of my favorite parts of yoga-meets-astrology. As the Sanskrit term *namasté* conveys, we are all one under the Sun.

5.2 Traditional Body–Zodiac Correlation

Leo: Spine

Also: Heart and hair (think of a lion's mane)

5.3 Wellness: Asana

Throughout time, people have considered the Sun to be the most visible form of divinity in our world. *Surya* refers to the Sun; temples honoring Surya exist all across India, and festivals are held each year to express gratitude for the Sun.

One way to express gratitude for our lives is by lavishing our bodies with loving care. Nurture the entire body by moving the spine in all five directions, every day: forward bend; back bend; inversion; twist to the right, twist to the left; side stretch (right and left).

Moving the spine in all five directions also pays tribute to the magnificent *sushumna nadi* (subtle-body energy channel) within the spine.

All yoga is good. For Leo, practice any asana (at any level, beginner to advanced, whatever is appropriate for you) while maintaining focus on the spine. You might try the following practices:

Simhasana, lion pose

Twist: *Pasasana*, noose pose

Back bend: *Ustrasana,* camel pose

Inversion: *Adho Mukha Vrksasana*, handstand pose

Forward bend: *Uttana Shishosana,* extended puppy pose

Side stretch: *Parivrtta Trikonasana,* revolved triangle pose

Surya Bhedana Pranayama, single nostril breath (Sun Piercing)

Featured Asana: *Surya Namaskar,* Salutation to the Sun

The devotional practice called Surya Namaskar may be performed at any time. This sequence of poses has several variations, some of which are quite rigorous. All follow a similar cyclical movement. Extend upward (like the rising Sun) and then bow down (like the setting Sun) to acknowledge an eternal cycle of light followed by darkness, followed by the return of light.

It is particularly auspicious to practice Surya Namaskar:

- Facing east (because the Sun rises in the east)
- At dawn
- With 108 repetitions

Do Surya Namaskar (or, if you're rushed, do one simple bow) to honor the Sun.

5.4 Exploration

At first glance, being yourself is the easiest thing in the world. Or it ought to be. After all, we have to be ourselves. How could it be otherwise?

As it turns out, there's more to the story.

The world is constantly trying to make us into something other than our simple, pure selves. Car manufacturers want us to drive, drive, drive.

And how about those sexy beer drinkers on the billboards? Home-improvement folks suggest the constant update of one's dreary abode. Beauty-product corporations and anti-aging industries urge us to be perpetually displeased with our hair, teeth, body size, age, shape, and eyelash color. And I'll confess my own weakness: svelte new yoga gear.

It's a full-time job keeping track of who we really are and what we genuinely want. It requires great courage to extract authenticity and purpose out of this thick and murky cultural soup.

5.5 Journaling

Ask yourself, "How have I been courageous?"

Make a list of the ways you currently are (or in the past have been) courageous. Please be very generous with yourself. Some days, getting out of bed is an act of courage. This I know.

Then try this visualization. Close your eyes and imagine a book. See the cover. Hold it, feel the binding. This is The Book of Your Life.

The cover is your cover: the chapters are phases of your life. Is it hardcover or paperback? How does the cover feel? Is there a picture on the cover?

Now carefully open the book and look inside. What does your book have to say? Spend some time imagining this. Then take a pen and write in The Book of Your Life.

5.6 Community

Lacey Fedel, Leo

To uphold the infamous Leo title of "King (or in my case Queen) of the Jungle," one must literally have a strong backbone both physically and spiritually.

I have an intense focus in my personal practice to open my spine deeper and deeper. As a teacher, I inform my students of the importance of keeping a strong and flexible spine.

Back bends, forward bends, side bends, and spine twisting feed the spine with fresh blood, oxygen, and nutrients. Connecting to the spine helps us to connect to all other areas of the body.

The spine holds ancient information: it is the bridge of the central nervous system. Every nerve, organ, gland, and system of the body communicates through the spine. Keeping the spine in good health is life insurance.

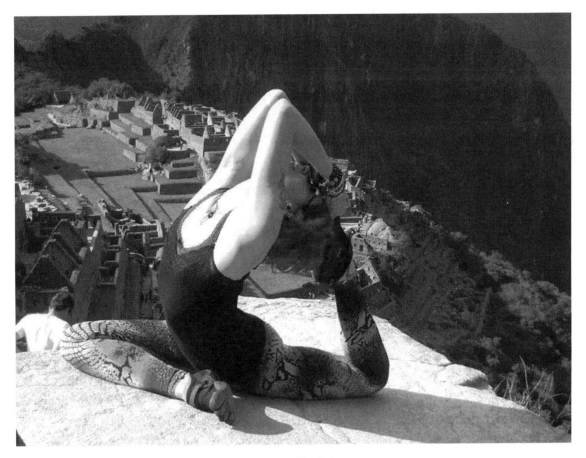

Lacey Fedel

5.7 Affirmation

I respect my courage.

To be yourself in a world that is constantly trying to make you something else is the greatest accomplishment.
-Emerson

I am sick and tired of everything but love.
-Rumi

6 virgo: ABDOMEN

Sun in Virgo: August 23 to September 22

Welcome to Virgo Yogastrology. This chapter encourages you to explore the wisdom of the sages, who claim that the moment you surrender, everything you have been wishing for is yours.

6.1 Element, Overview, Ruling Planet: Mercury

6.2 Traditional Body–Zodiac Correlation: Abdomen

6.3 Wellness: Asanas

6.4 Exploration: Now, I Surrender

6.5 Journaling: What would you like to surrender?

6.6 Community: Faith Hunter, Virgo; and Sara LeVere, Virgo

6.7 Affirmation: I let go of that which does not serve the Highest Good.

The gift of Virgo, the Goddess of Sweet Grain, and twisting poses is surrender. Let go of what no longer serves you–make room for the new.

6.1 Virgo Element, Overview, Ruling Planet

Whoever created the hackneyed depiction of Virgo as sexless, critical, and cold, with spectacles pushed down his nose, please step forward. I beg to differ. In my opinion, whoever wrote that description does not know Virgo. Here's the real deal.

Well-developed Virgos care deeply about doing things well, in a healthy way. Notice I said "well," not right. That keen Virgo intellect knows there is not just one way to do something. There are countless ways. Yes, Virgo has done his research, and done it very well.

Well-developed Virgos know. What might feel like criticism is actually friendly advice: Virgo usually knows how to make things turn out well. From commandeering a boardroom to cleaning the bathroom, you can count on Virgo. Do what it takes to please Virgo, and you might find you've got the sweetest, smartest, funniest, and most loyal–did I mention modest?–friend for life.

Earth sign Virgo's symbol is the Goddess of Sweet Grain (also known as the Virgin Goddess). This goddess represents how some of the sweetest, most useful things in life simply reveal themselves.

The Virgin Goddess is holding a sheaf of grain, representing the harvest. The wheat has been separated from the chaff, revealing the sweet grains. Who would ingest chaff? Anyone who tried would find it inedible. The fine skill of discernment is a matter of paying attention, noticing what works, and tuning in to what's happening. The goddess encourages us to go with what works. She accepts the sweetest grains; she feasts on them every day. It's only natural.

Nature is on your side. Mother Nature is an intelligent teacher.

Ruling planet: Mercury

Mercury rules two zodiac signs, Gemini and Virgo.

In Gemini, Mercury is at its speedy and fact-finding best, zipping about, collecting data, amassing storehouses of fun facts. Mercury Gemini knows something about everything. We're talking quantity, not quality, for Gemini Mercury.

In Virgo, Mercury is more discriminating and analytical. There is depth in Virgo, coupled with considerable intellect, and this incites one to discern the truly useful from useless riff-raff.

Digest what is useful; surrender or let go of that which has no use. Quality, not quantity, for Virgo Mercury.

Some astrologers suggest that Chiron, not Mercury, is the true ruler of Virgo—or at least an appropriate co-ruler. Most astrologers agree that Chiron is a sensitive, vulnerable point in an astrology chart. This planetoid (mini-planet), or asteroid, was discovered in 1977. Upon its discovery, a new astrological era was born.

Because of its location in the sky, Chiron is sometimes called "the Rainbow Bridge" (Barbara Hand Clow has written a book by that title, which you may want to check out). This bridge is an energetic force between many features of life—bridging, for example, human consciousness (represented by planets visible to the naked eye) and the unconscious realm (represented by planets not visible); the past (antiquity, status quo, Saturn) and the future (the new era we are challenged to create, innovation, Uranus); and more.

Chiron, also known as the Wounded Healer, represents coming to terms with sensitivity and vulnerability.

One can develop the capacity for empathy as well as ignite a profound gift of healing by becoming intimate with Chiron and what it represents.

Helping others heal is the silver lining of Chiron, the Wounded Healer.

6.2 Traditional Body–Zodiac Correlation

Virgo: Abdomen

Also: Small intestine and gall bladder

6.3 Wellness: Asanas

A magnificent system of digestion takes place in the human body; specifically, in the abdomen.

Three steps are involved:

- Taking in nutrients
- Digesting or assimilation
- Surrendering or releasing

6 VIRGO: ABDOMEN

The cycle of taking in, assimilation, and surrender or releasing–whether it's food, or life experiences–is a complex process. It requires keen discrimination. When functioning well, our digestive system keeps us fed and happy, allowing us to take in goodies and release that which does not serve us, and that clears space for the cycle to begin anew.

When we do poses that emphasize the abdomen, we may feel calm or we may be moved in a deep way. The abdomen is a very sensitive area of the body. It can be fascinating to witness what comes up when it's stimulated. Just watch, without judging.

All yoga is good. For Virgo, practice any asana (at any level, beginner to advanced, whatever is appropriate for you) while maintaining focus on the abdomen. You might try the following practices:

Bhujangasana, cobra pose

Mayurasana, peacock pose

Marichyasana, the sage's pose

Paripurna Navasana, full boat pose

Uddiyana Bandha, upward abdominal lock

Parivrtta Parsvakonasana, revolved side angle pose

Parivrtta Janu Sirsasana, revolved head-to-knee pose

Featured Asana: *Bharadvajasana,* seated twisting pose (or do a very simple seated twist; see 6.5 below).

Before you practice your twisting pose, ask yourself what you'd like to let go of, what you want to surrender. Jot down a few notes about this.

Then do a twisting pose and see what comes up for you.

6.4 Exploration

I've heard all about surrender. Several popular spiritual teachers talk about it, and they highly recommend it. I've taught my yoga students about surrender (with twisting poses, usually).

Still, sometimes I find myself hedging my bets.

There have been moments when I've caught a glimpse of this thought streaming along, deep inside me: "After I get this done, I'll surrender. Once that bill is paid, I'll let go and trust how the universe is unfolding. After I finish this page, I'll release my limitations and align with divine will."

It's a funny trick that I play on myself. I know I can't surrender later.

If I'm ever going to do it, it has to happen now, not later. The only time we have to surrender is the only time there is. That time is now.

6.5 Journaling

The sages say that the moment we surrender, everything we have been wishing for is ours.

Let's explore an embodied experience of surrender. Please note, *this works only if you do it*; you can't just read about it and expect to get results.

Try this simple seated twist. You can do this one seated in a chair, or on the floor in *Sukhasana* (easy cross-legged pose).

1. Place right-hand fingertips on the floor, near your right hip; if you're sitting in a chair that has arms, grasp the right-side arm (or seat) of the chair with your right hand.

2. Cross left arm in front of your torso—left hand to right knee; inhale, elongate spine up; gently draw navel toward spine.

3. Exhale. Use your arms to help twist the lower abdomen to the right. Stay firmly seated and twist only the lower abdomen (do not twist the shoulders or neck; the tendency here is to skip the abdomen and crank the neck).

4. Inhale and extend the spine upward gently, and on the exhalation, continue to twist only the lower abdomen to the right (stay firmly seated); remain in this focused phase of the pose (in other words, don't twist the upper torso) and breathe.

5. On an inhalation, elongate spine up; release any tension in shoulders and neck, face, and jaw and move into your full expression of the

pose by twisting your upper torso, shoulders, neck, and head as far as is comfortable, to the right.

6. Continue with focusing breathing; when you're ready, on an exhalation, release the twist; return to center, pause, and breathe.

7. Repeat on the second side (follow steps 1. – 6. and twist to the left).

Blissful sensations arise when ida and pingala (nadis or energy channels on either side of the sushumna nadi in the spine) cross one another, as they do in twisting poses such as this one.

Describe the experience you had twisting. What let go, for you?

What would you like to surrender?

6.6 Community

Faith Hunter, Virgo

> When I feel stressed or worried, I immediately get an uncomfortable sensation in my abdomen.
>
> This is a clear signal that I need to surrender and let go.
>
> When I surrender, not only does my body feel better, but things in life flow with ease.

6 VIRGO: ABDOMEN

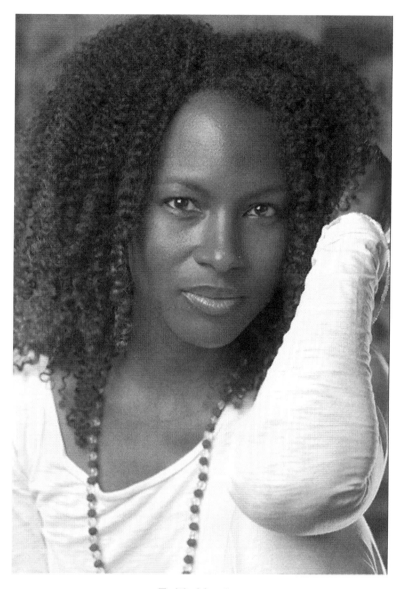

Faith Hunter

Sara LeVere, Virgo

The abdomen is such a special part of our body. It houses vital organs as well as our capacity for digestion, filtration of food and toxins, and digestion of information.

What do we choose to digest in life? What do we choose to let pass through?

The abdomen is a powerful guide; it contains a mass of electrical impulses with more nerve cells than the brain. That "gut" feeling or "butterflies-in-the-stomach" experience is a physical response to what we intuitively feel or know. If ever you are unsure about something, ask your guide. Your abdomen always will guide you to the honest truth about what is right for you.

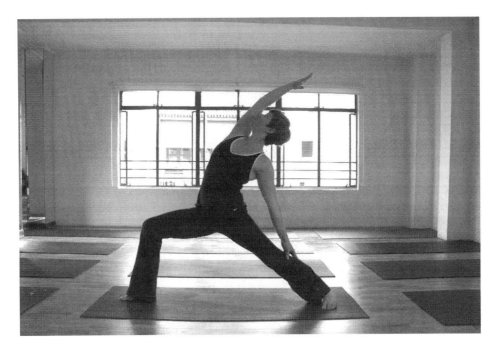

Sara LeVere

6.7 Affirmation

I let go of that which does not serve the Highest Good.

> *It is not by resisting or running away from, but by that deep act of surrender that the divine is realized. And that amazingly does not take time. Surrender can only be now.*
> *-Eckhart Tolle*

7 libra: LOWER BACK

Sun in Libra: September 23 to October 22

Welcome to Libra Yogastrology. This chapter invites you to explore solitude and partnership, and journal about what really matters to you.

7.1 Element, Overview, Ruling Planet: Venus
7.2 Traditional Body–Zodiac Correlation: Lower Back
7.3 Wellness: Asanas
7.4 Exploration: Partner Poses Teach Presence
7.5 Journaling: Would you like to partner up?
7.6 Community: Tiffany Cruikshank, Libra; and Elena Brower, Libra
7.7 Affirmation: I give freely and receive plentifully.

If you're with a partner today, may you both enjoy good company. And if you're solo, may you revel in your own good company.

7.1 Libra Element, Overview, Ruling Planet

The symbol for air sign Libra is the scales. This is the only sign of the zodiac with an inanimate object (neither animal nor human) for a symbol, but that doesn't make gracious Libra any less humane.

In fact, some would say Libra is the most humane, cordial, and sociable sign in the zodiac. For Libra, life is all about social grace, putting others at ease, and balance.

The greatest balancing act in our lives is between self and others. Libra devotes himself to the fine art of interpersonal relationship. He often has a sixth sense about what other people need and want, sometimes even before the other person knows what he wants.

The exceptionally diplomatic Libra can be highly effective as a negotiator or strategist. With so much charm and harmonious energy, what's not to like about gracious, beautiful Libra?

Ruling planet: Venus

Venus rules two zodiac signs: Taurus and Libra. In Taurus, Venus luxuriates in the physical realm. She loves monetary wealth and gourmet cuisine, scented body oils, and long days spent soaking up goodies at a spa. Sensual pleasures are paramount to voluptuous Venus in Taurus.

In Libra, Venus is partial to the finery. Nothing crude will do; it offends her delicate sensibilities.

Libra Venus lives on the high side of life: Art. Education. Gorgeous poetry. High-quality, professional musicianship. Witty repartee and creative ideas inspire ever-tasteful Venus in Libra.

7.2 Traditional Body–Zodiac Correlation

Libra: Lower back

Also: Kidneys

7.3 Wellness: Asanas

One of the main components of overall health and wellness in the body–and well-being of the lower back, in particular–involves the sacrum, the big bone in your lower back. The word "sacrum" comes from Latin and Greek roots meaning sacred.

Consider these qualities of the sacrum:

- It is in close proximity to the procreative organs.
- The first three chakras in the subtle body are situated around the sacrum.
- The sacrum is gender dimorphic; it's shaped differently in males than in females.

All yoga is good. For Libra, practice any asana (at any level, beginner to advanced, whatever is appropriate for you) while maintaining focus on the lower back. You might try the following practices:

Sphinx, baby back bend

Salabasana, locust pose

Parsva Bakasana, side crane pose

Natarajasana, lord of the dance pose

Ardha Uttanasana, standing half forward bend

Ardha Matsyendrasana, half lord of the fishes pose

Adho Mukha Svanasana, downward-facing dog pose

Featured Asana: *Natarajasana,* lord of the dance pose

Natarajasana is a much-loved balance pose that can help us maintain balance in yoga practice, and in life—which can be tricky.

Here are three ways to stay balanced and feel good in your body and in your life.

1. Stand on one foot.

Balance on one foot and reach out, touch the wall. This simple technique reminds you how nourishing it is to accept support.

Accept support. Ask a friend or family member to listen while you vent for five minutes. Offer to do the same for him or her.

2. Do balance poses.

Balance poses (which can be as simple as standing on one foot, or as demanding as poses such as *Eka Pada Koundiyanasana II*) bring the right and left sides of your body into harmony.

Harmonize your body's rhythms with the pulse of nature. Get up with the Sun at dawn. Go to bed early.

3. Take ten.

Ten minutes a day, spent in an activity that you love, can completely uplift you.

Every day, take at least ten minutes to do something–such as practicing yoga, listening to music, or taking a walk–that leaves you feeling balanced and refreshed.

7.4 Exploration

If you like partner poses, spend time connecting with your lover, a friend, a special child, or your yoga classmates, and do fun partner poses.

Closeness and trust happen naturally when we touch one another and experience nonverbal intimacy. Touch and intimacy deepen our connection with ourselves, as well as with others.

You can discover a lot about your capacity to give—and at the same time, fine-tune your ability to take good care of yourself—when you do partner poses.

You learn about receiving, too, which is a very special skill. Partner poses teach us how to be thoroughly present while we let someone give to us.

7.5 Journaling

Do you enjoy partner poses? Why, or why not? What's your preference: partner poses or a solo yoga practice?

In your day-to-day life, do you love spending time alone, or are you the sort of person who enjoys partnering up whenever you can? Does your relationship-life feel balanced? Release any judgments. It's all good.

7.6 Community

Tiffany Cruikshank, Libra

> Balance is crucial both on and off the mat. The perfect balance of passion and purpose, masculine and feminine, yin and yang, is the source of health and happiness.

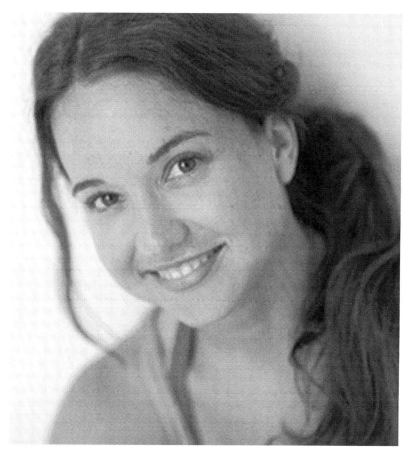

Tiffany Cruikshank

Elena Brower, Libra

I am always playing with balance. The balance of giving and receiving is elusive, and it informs everything I do, from coaching, to teaching yoga, to parenting. It's a practice.

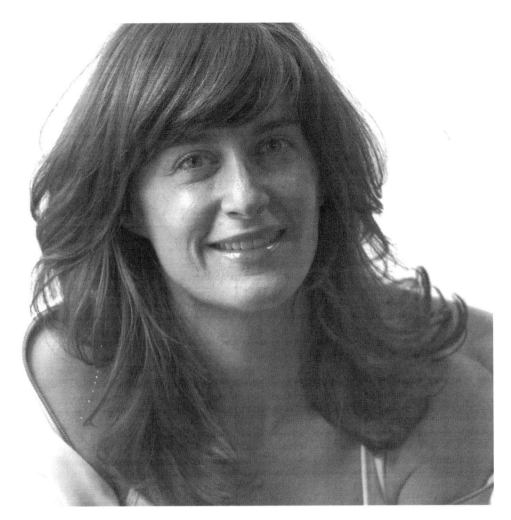

Elena Brower

7.7 Affirmation

I give freely and receive plentifully.

> *We live only to discover beauty.*
> *All else is a form of waiting.*
> *-Kahlil Gibran*

8 scorpio: PELVIS

Sun in Scorpio: October 23 to November 21

Welcome to Scorpio Yogastrology. This chapter invites you to explore the magic of transformation and indulge in a little creative Bedtimeasana.

8.1 Element, Overview, Ruling Planet: Pluto

8.2 Traditional Body–Zodiac Correlation: Pelvis

8.3 Wellness: Asanas

8.4 Exploration: Bedtimeasana

8.5 Journaling: What was the most transformative period of your life?

8.6 Community: Sadie Nardini, Scorpio

8.7 Affirmation: I live an authentic, empowered life.

In this chapter we will practice a traditional gesture: *Chin mudra.* Subtly and powerfully, this mudra expresses an intense, purposeful intent to invoke transformation.

8.1 Scorpio Element, Overview, Ruling Planet

Scorpio is a water sign, and it's the most intense, passionate, and determined water sign of all. Quite possibly, Scorpio is the most intense sign in the zodiac.

Traits include a fierce determination to triumph against all odds, ruthlessness when pursuing a goal, and extreme emotions. Scorpio possesses an intuitive, mysterious, secretive, and highly sexual nature. Be aware: He can be vengeful and treacherous. And at the same time, he can be the most loyal, deeply devoted friend.

Two animals—the scorpion and the eagle—as well as the mythological creature known as the phoenix are associated with Scorpio.

Scorpion: Crawling on the ground, seeking out hidden spaces, scorpions are at home in the low-lying, dark realms of the world. When provoked, the scorpion will strike with a vengeance. This is Scorpio's dark side.

Eagle: The wings of the bird take Scorpio far above earthly limitations. From their lofty perspective, eagles see a world that others may never see. This is the high side of Scorpio.

Phoenix: The mythological phoenix is an immortal bird that rises from its own ashes to make a remarkable comeback, to be born anew. He knows both sides: light and dark, creation and destruction. The phoenix transcends the two extremes. It is a symbol of transformation.

Ruling planet: Pluto

Since its discovery in 1930, Pluto (now considered a dwarf planet) has been the planetary ruler of this intense and intriguing zodiac sign, Scorpio.

Pluto, in an astrology chart, shows an area of life where one might face relentless cycles of creation, demise, and reconstruction.

According to Pluto, we possess an undeniable power to transform our lives and ignite fresh *joie de vivre*. See Pluto as an ally who urges or perhaps forces you to be reborn, to become a more empowered person.

8.2 Traditional Body–Zodiac Correlation

Scorpio: Pelvis

Also: Genitals, reproductive organs, urinary tract, and bladder

8.3 Wellness: Asanas

Think of how often we gesture with our hands. Waving at a friend. The ubiquitous handshake. Holding hands with our loved ones.

Chin mudra is an ancient traditional gesture for the hands, symbolizing the interconnectedness of human consciousness and supreme consciousness.

Touch the tip of your thumb with the tip of your index finger. Allow the other three fingers to point down gently toward the earth. Open your palm in a gesture of receptivity.

In Chin mudra, an unbroken circle is formed by the index finger and the thumb. The circle represents the true goal of yoga–union, or oneness, merging the individual with the universal. Also, the circle forms a circuit, allowing potent energy that would otherwise dissipate into the environment to remain in your body.

All yoga is good. For Scorpio, practice any asana (at any level, beginner to advanced, whatever is appropriate for you) while maintaining focus on the pelvis. You might try the following practices:

Dandasana, staff pose

Ustrasana, camel pose

Padmasana, lotus pose

Malasana, garland pose

Janu Sirsasana, head-to-knee forward bend

Upavistha Konasana, wide-angle seated forward bend

Dwi Pada Viparita Dandasana, upward facing two-foot staff pose

Featured Asana: *Baddha Konasana,* cobbler pose, bound angle pose

Put your hands in Chin mudra in Baddha Konasana. Place your hands on or near your bent knees to stimulate an energy channel (called a nadi) running from the knees, up the inner thighs, into the pelvis. Hello, Scorpio.

8.4 Exploration

One of the best places on the planet to do yoga is not Costa Rica or New Zealand. Don't get me wrong, I love this beautiful planet. But truly, one of the best places in the whole world to do yoga is right down the hall. That's right, your bedroom.

More specifically, your bed. Stay with me here.

You're in your bedroom for several hours a day (or night).

So do yoga there, and get in a daily practice no matter what, even if it becomes your nightly practice.

And the room is full of props. Pillows and blankets make cozy yoga props, and your bed makes a comfortable surface for practicing. Keep the lighting soft, the room quiet and private. It's great to have the yoga vibe everywhere—especially in your bedroom.

You are invited to do Bedtimeasana now—feel free to invent a pose that's just right for you. Gather props, cushions, your eye pillow, whatever makes you feel comfortable. Let Bedtimeasana be extra nice: Set up your own super-comfy bedtime yoga pose.

If you don't want to invent a pose, do *Shavasana*; it's a great bedtime pose.

If you get creative and invent a new pose, sketch it. Give it a name. Do Bedtimeasana poses every night, if you can. And if you decide to make your own Bedtime Yoga DVD, let me know. Sweet dreams.

8.5 Journaling

Ask yourself, "What was the most transformative period in my life?"

Look back: "When was that extremely transformative period?"

Look within: "Who have I become as a result of that transformation; how has my life changed?"

Look forward: "How would I like to transform in the future?"

8.6 Community

Sadie Nardini, Scorpio

> I am passionate. Adventurous. Always seeking (and leading) toward personal growth, psycho—I mean psychic. I was born on the Scorpio–Sagittarius cusp, and I love to travel.
>
> I think the traditional body–zodiac correlation resonates quite strongly, based on the fact that this is the first time I've seen the body–zodiac

correlations, and my specialties are pelvic and lumbar core anatomy, and transformative breath-work in the vinyasa flow.

I live and (literally) breathe transformation and transmutation.

I teach Patanjali's Three Steps to Transformation, Kriya Yoga, and I believe that we as yogis can work the alchemy of our realizations about our true nature through–and into–real-world actions like shifting the breath, refining all our movements on and off the mat, listening to the guidance of our ruling planets, watching closely for the teachings and signs that are all around us, and being courageous enough to trust what we hear from inside and out.

As a Scorpio–Sagittarius cusp with five planets in Scorpio, beyond my Sun in Scorpio, I love the mystical and the practical perspectives that aligning with astrology brings into my life. I've found that it explains a lot about me from day to day, and I make sure to consult my horoscope(s) daily just to remain in alignment with the greater forces around me.

Why not believe in magic wherever we can?

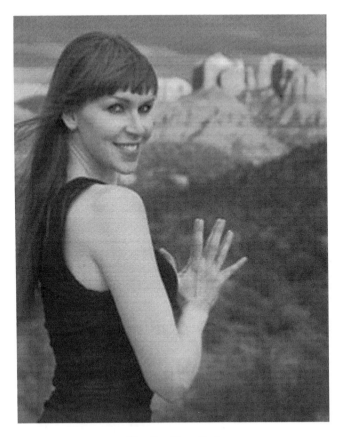

Sadie Nardini

8.7 Affirmation

I live an authentic, empowered life.

We do practices to get through life—alive!
-Krishna Das

Without accepting the fact that everything changes,
we cannot find perfect composure.
-Shunryu Suzuki

9 sagittarius: HIPS

Sun in Sagittarius: November 22 to December 21

Welcome to Sagittarius Yogastrology. This chapter takes you on a pilgrimage to the most sacred temple in the world (it's closer than you think).

9.1 Element, Overview, Ruling Planet: Jupiter

9.2 Traditional Body–Zodiac Correlation: Hips

9.3 Wellness: Asanas

9.4 Exploration: Hanuman

9.5 Journaling: What was the most memorable journey you've ever taken?

9.6 Community: Shakti Sunfire, Sagittarius

9.7 Affirmation: I let my body love what it loves.

Yoga creates an unparalleled sense of freedom in your body–and that translates into freedom in your life. Enjoy the adventure.

9.1 Aries Element, Overview, Ruling Planet

Fire sign Sagittarius: The philosopher and the pilgrim, the adventurer and the optimist. Filled with faith, Sagittarius tends to do things in a big way (perhaps that explains why the big Thanksgiving Day feast is held at this time of year). Sagittarius is an exciting catalyst for anything big and new.

You'll find the Sagittarius streak (in yourself, and in your friends, teachers, and role models) drawn to do vision quests, try bungee jumping, learn more and more about everything, and take the hero's journey. And then Sagittarius usually likes to teach what he has learned to others, or in some way expand upon it even more.

The only trouble is the occasional delusion of grandeur (although Sagittarius may not be delusional at all–listen up because what he's talking about may be the next Big Deal in everyone's life).

Two of the symbols for Sagittarius–the archer, and his arrow–symbolize movement. And in Yogastrology, we associate this sign with the ancient tradition of pilgrimage, a devotional journey taken by a seeker; it's a grand voyage with a particular intention.

Sagittarians tend to be dauntless truth seekers who love exploration and adventure, long-distance travel, and spirituality. All of us can learn from this sign. Sagittarius lives life as a magnificent adventure.

Ruling planet: Jupiter

Jupiter is the largest planet; it has more mass than all the other planets combined. Astrologically, Jupiter signifies expansion, good will, and good fortune.

Of course, even with Jupiter, we can't simply kick back and wait for blessings to shower down upon us (although, with Jupiter, they may). And Jupiter does tend to make a person exceptionally optimistic, squandering resources with the belief that there's always more where that came from (which usually there is).

One thing you can count on: Jupiter always provides clues about when and where opportunities for expansion may pour in. When Jupiter is present, your job is to take advantage of the opportunities that come your way.

This inspiring planet encourages leaps of faith; its influence takes us on big adventures and leads us toward our higher calling. Jovial Jupiter is an indicator of prosperity and an espouser of wisdom. Forever inviting experiences and ideas, fascinated by new cultures and people, always introducing more color and spice, Jupiter has the Midas touch.

9.2 Traditional Body–Zodiac Correlation

Sagittarius: Hips

Also: Sciatic nerve, thighs, and buttocks

9.3 Wellness: Asanas

Your body is a temple. Close your eyes, and listen within. What do you hear in the inner sanctum, in the temple of your body?

If you're like most people, one of the things you hear is your tight hips kvetching your daily jog, weekly ski trip, or the simple fact of sitting all day at a desk, then driving home, followed by taking a seat at the dining-room table.

All yoga is good. For Sagittarius, practice any asana (at any level, beginner to advanced, whatever is appropriate for you) while maintaining focus on the hips. You might try the following practices:

Camatkarasana, wild thing

Utthan Pristhasana, lizard pose

Agnistambhasana, fire log pose

Anantasana, side-reclining leg lift

Ananda Balasana, happy baby pose

Eka Pada Raja Kapotasana, half pigeon pose

Supta Baddha Konasana, reclining bound angle pose

Featured Asana: *Anjaneyasana,* lunge pose

After your hip-opener asana practice, revisit this and take note of what has shifted. Your body is a temple. Close your eyes, and listen within. What do you hear in the inner sanctum, in the temple of your body?

9.4 Exploration

Who would name a yoga pose after his or her mother? The Lord of Yoga, that's who.

The lunge pose, *Anjaneyasana,* is named after Anjaney.

Her famous son, Hanuman, is the Lord of Yoga, the very embodiment of physical strength. He also possesses a big heart and is a model of devotion.

The Lord of Yoga is honored by millions in India. Many temples exist to worship him, and devotees make regular pilgrimages there. They ask Hanuman to remove their suffering and to fulfill their wishes.

We're on a pilgrimage to a Hanuman temple. What suffering will you ask Hanuman to remove?

What wishes will you ask Hanuman to fulfill?

The grace of Hanuman, the Lord of Yoga, lives inside your heart. May all suffering be removed. May all your wishes be fulfilled.

9.5 Journaling

Ask yourself, "Of all the journeys I've taken, what is the most memorable?"

What was your intention when you planned that journey?

Are you taking a journey in the future? What is your destination? Your intention?

Do you have a devotional haven, a special place of pilgrimage?

Your place of pilgrimage may be halfway around the world. Or it could be your meditation room down the hall. Perhaps best of all, your destination may be inside you…a pilgrimage to your heart.

9.6 Community

Shakti Sunfire, Sagittarius

> I have nearly all of my planets in fiery Sagittarius and truly resonate with the wandering gypsy nature of this sign and the influence of expansive Jupiter.
>
> I am all about experience and knowledge, especially when it comes to the unseen world, where I dive head-first into various philosophies from many traditions. I devour books, speak multiple languages, and am home no more than I am away. Freedom is my middle name, and as the eternal optimist, I provoke my fair share of celebration.

I do hula hoop for a living if that says anything (about the traditional body–zodiac correlation for Sagittarius, the hips)! More than that, I love to dance in general. I also find deep hip openers to be the juiciest work I can do on a yoga mat.

I am always on the move, driven more than anything else to follow the pilgrimage of my own heart's desire.

Everywhere I go I seek holy places where spirit is engaged and truly honored. From Mother Teresa's tomb in Calcutta, India to the Black Madonna of Montserrat in Barcelona, Spain to the Belly Button of the Moon in Tulum, Mexico, I dedicate my life to walking the path of self-realization and inner knowing.

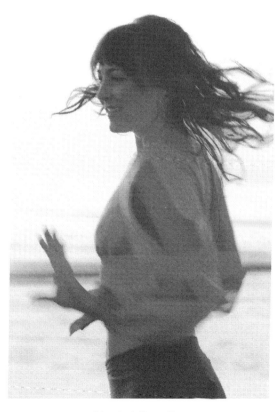

Shakti Sunfire

9.7 Affirmation

I let my body love what it loves.

Come, come, whoever you are. Wonderer, worshipper, lover of leaving.
It doesn't matter. Ours is not a caravan of despair.
Come, even if you have broken your vow a thousand times.
Come, yet again, come, come.
-Rumi

10 capricorn: KNEES

Sun in Capricorn: December 22 to January 20

Welcome to Capricorn Yogastrology. This chapter encourages you to explore the timeless wisdom and taste the sweet fruit of dharmic action.

10.1 Element, Overview, Ruling Planet: Saturn

10.2 Traditional Body–Zodiac Correlation: Knees

10.3 Wellness: Asanas

10.4 Exploration: Dharma, the Wisdom of the Ages

10.5 Journaling: To whom (or what) are you committed?

10.6 Community: Laurèn Rovira, Capricorn

10.7 Affirmation: I embrace dharma with commitment, compassion, and contentment.

What image comes up for you when you hear the word *dharma* (the Sanskrit term for righteousness or right action)? You will have the opportunity to explore dharma and experience its rich rewards.

10.1 Capricorn Element, Overview, Ruling Planet

It is said that earth sign Capricorn's symbol, the mountain goat, can ascend higher than can any other mammal. He does this by being sure-footed and steadfast.

Steadfastness in human form means staying in alignment with values such as commitment. Goethe said, "Concerning all acts of initiative and creation, there is one elementary truth the ignorance of which kills countless ideas and splendid plans: The moment one definitely commits oneself, then Providence moves too. All sorts of things occur to help one that would never otherwise have occurred."

Commitment pays high dividends. Another side (which may be exhibited when Capricorn is not fully developed): Capricorn can be a wee bit inhibited. But in most cases, this sign is resourceful, loyal, committed, compassionate, and content.

Ruling planet: Saturn

Saturn represents limitations. As the last planet that can be seen with the naked eye, Saturn defines an outer limit of our universe. Its influence represents that which is held in place and defined (remember the rings around Saturn).

Hard lessons and perhaps some fears show up here, too. That's Saturn's down side.

The up side is this: Drawing boundaries works. Demarcation is very effective. So while Saturn may seem daunting or repressive at times, the influence of this planet can eliminate what's not working, clarify what is working, and lend support by making the best things in life last.

Saturn imparts structure and stability in an otherwise amorphous world. From Saturn, we learn about taking responsibility and honoring our commitments. Teachers, authorities, and father figures–replete with their rules and regulations, the disciplinary actions they impose, and the fear they might engender–are Saturnian. Although not always pleasant, the influence of this planet does help us grow.

A Saturn Return happens for everyone around age twenty-nine, and again around age fifty-eight, when transiting Saturn returns to its natal location. At these times you can make significant course corrections and get back on track.

This planet's influence imparts genuine maturity, making you stronger and more capable of handling fear.

Eventually, Saturn becomes your shining jewel. Like a teacher, mentor, or parental figure who really cares, Saturn influences your life for the better.

10.2 Traditional Body–Zodiac Correlation

Capricorn: Knees

Also: Skeleton, bones, and teeth

10.3 Wellness: Asana

Doing yoga can bring up many feelings. When the knees are involved, fear can come up, especially the fear of moving forward. Let's explore what it's like to have a strong, loving, and fertile relationship between yoga and fear.

Yoga empowers a gradual awakening. The process begins with a willingness to slow down, pause, and apply the sweet, soft balm of time. Then you can make the choice to befriend yourself, to stay with whatever bubbles up inside. Stay focused, listen to inner messages. Attuned to your inner voice, allow yourself to be guided into a tender embrace with wounded, fearful parts of yourself. In this embrace, it is possible to transform fear into love.

Make a commitment to yoga, and compassion will be there to help uproot fear.

Release fear, and gentle waves of contentment will wash over you.

At this time, come to your knees (such as in a kneeling pose) and offer gratitude for *everything*. Even things that are...troubling? Especially offer gratitude for things that trouble you, for those things expose your vulnerabilities, which in turn open the portal to transformation. Apply awareness, practice gratitude–and commitment, compassion, and contentment–and vulnerabilities become strengths.

All yoga is good. For Capricorn, practice any asana (at any level, beginner to advanced, whatever is appropriate for you) while maintaining focus on the knees. You might try the following practices:

Virasana, hero pose

Utkatasana, chair pose

Pasasana, noose pose

Parighasana, gate pose

Tadasana, mountain pose

Virabhadrasana, warrior pose

Baddha Konasana, cobbler pose, bound angle pose

Featured Asana: *Vrksasana,* tree pose

In tree pose, imagine roots extending down, from your knee to the sole of your standing foot, into the earth. Like the tree's roots, reach down to receive stability, support, and nourishment from the earth.

Extend your arms upward, as the limbs of the tree reach toward the heavens to soak up sunshine. Reach up, from the raised (bent) knee all the way up to and through your fingertips, to receive genuine inspiration and higher intelligence from above.

Yoga embodies the union of heaven and earth.

10.4 Exploration

Like the ancient Chinese Tao, dharma refers to a natural flow and absolute justice.

Explore the three C's of dharma—commitment, compassion, contentment—within yourself, in your practice, and in your life.

Embody dharma. Let dharma become increasingly real for you; allow this ancient wisdom to reveal its riches.

Notice the precious moments when you sense pervasive order, beauty, and balance; when you are aware that everything is in harmony and you breathe a sigh of relief; when you are genuinely content. In these moments, you are experiencing dharma.

Brihadaranyaka Upanishad (describing dharma): Original Truth…natural harmony, and the purest of all reality.

10.5 Journaling

The three C's of dharma are commitment, compassion, and contentment.

- Commitment: To whom or what are you committed?
- Compassion: How does compassion show up in your life?
- Contentment: Where do you find the greatest contentment?

Imagine yourself experiencing more and more contentment. Now make up a symbol that represents you basking in lavish contentment. You are the goddess (or god) of complete contentment.

10.6 Community

Laurèn Rovira, Capricorn

I am immensely grateful, which involves kneeling and bowing in grace.

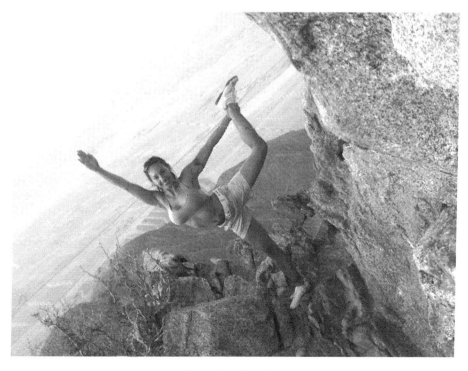

Laurèn Rovira

10.7 Affirmation

I embrace dharma: commitment, compassion, contentment.

Here is a test to find if your mission on earth is finished.
If you're alive, it isn't.
-Richard Bach

Going back to Saturn where the rings all glow.
Rainbow, moonbeams, and orange snow.
On Saturn people live to be two hundred and five.
-Stevie Wonder

11 aquarius: ANKLES

Sun in Aquarius: January 21 to February 18

Welcome to Aquarius Yogastrology. This chapter introduces the primordial lovers, Shiva and Shakti. Experience their embrace and sip this bliss for yourself.

11.1 Element, Overview, Ruling Planets: Saturn and Uranus

11.2 Traditional Body–Zodiac Correlation: Ankles

11.3 Wellness: Asanas

11.4 Exploration: Shiva, Shakti, and Bliss

11.5 Journaling: How do you embody unity?

11.6 Community: Leah Kim, Aquarius

11.7 Affirmation: I practice radical self-acceptance.

Shiva and Shakti are the primordial lovers. Some say the entire practice of yoga is for the purpose of reuniting these lovers...or to have the realization that they are inescapably linked in all ways and forever.

11.1 Aquarius Element, Overview, Ruling Planets

Up in the sky, embedded in the heavenly constellation for air sign Aquarius, we find the symbol for this sign—a human figure pouring cool water from a jug.

Aquarians can be cool, even aloof. Their impersonal side relates to their intense focus on tribal affiliations and the social codes that bind a society together (think Saturn).

Couple this with the Aquarian revolutionary zeal that dismantles outdated societal codes (a trait of zealous Uranus), and we find Aquarian visionaries introducing progressive change into the structure of society.

Starting off with a bang, we find Uranus and Saturn, co-rulers of Aquarius, engaged in a stormy love-hate relationship. You cannot imagine two entities any more different. What brings them together? Do opposites attract?

Ruling planets: Saturn and Uranus

Saturn: The teacher, the taskmaster. Father Time. Saturn rules tradition and the establishment, representing the past and maturity. Saturn pins things down. This planet represents the instinct to commit. Stable, conservative Saturn maintains long-term social structures.

Nothing can last without the Saturnian influence. And Saturn is head instructor for Reality 101; he teaches responsibility and the value of tenacity, tough love, and sacrifice. Work hard. The job may be tedious, especially because Saturn depends entirely upon Uranus for fresh inspiration—but diligence is beautifully rewarded in the end.

Uranus: Freedom lover. Radical genius. The great awakener. Uranus represents the future and youthfulness. When you see a zap of lightning, think Uranus; this planet rules electricity.

Unexpected, unannounced, the influence of Uranus sweeps in and shatters whatever has outlived its purpose, making way for the new. Trailblazing Uranus hurls laser beams of truth, laced with a brilliant eccentricity. This planet presides over inspiration and innovation, even genius.

Caveat: Uranian revolution must collude with Saturn's discipline to bring about lasting change.

11.2 Traditional Body–Zodiac Correlation

Aquarius : Ankles

Also: Lower legs and the bioelectrical system

11.3 Wellness: Asanas

Meet the primordial lovers, Shiva and Shakti.

Shakti is matter, movement, and energy. Nothing gets done when she's not around (imagine that).

Shiva is formlessness…silence. I mean really, what can you say about Shiva?

Nothing exists that is not Shiva.

Ultimately, Shiva and Shakti are not two separate entities; they are inextricably intertwined, always and forever, in their lovers' dance. They cannot not be, for they are one. They're two sides of one complete being. We simply cannot have one without the other. Their inseparable embrace–their eternal dance–creates the universe.

Shiva and Shakti show us the inescapable link between life's opposites. It's easy to see this duality in these pairs:

- Up–Down
- Light–Dark
- Empty–Full

The list of pairs goes on and on. What comes to your mind when you reflect on pairs of opposites?

In yoga practice, we practice asana on the right side of the body, then the left side (or vice versa), which is a direct embodied experience of the pairs of opposites. Also the practice soothes the mind by harmonizing communication between the right and left hemispheres of the brain (via the bridge between these two brain hemispheres, the corpus callosum).

All yoga is good. For Aquarius, practice any asana (at any level, beginner to advanced, whatever is appropriate for you) while maintaining focus on the ankles. You might try the following practices:

Padmasana, lotus pose

Malasana, garland pose

Garudasana, eagle pose

Krounchasana, heron pose

Viparita Karani, legs up the wall pose

Supta Padangusthasana, reclining big toe pose

Parivrtta Parsvakonasana, revolved side angle pose

Featured Asana: *Balasana*, child's pose, is restful and invigorating at the same time. This pose is much more potent than it looks—and it can be done on its own or sequenced between more intense asanas.

11.4 Exploration

Stop. Get a glass of water and a spoon. This is important. Bring the water and spoon back here. Do it. You'll see why. I'll wait for you.

Got your water and a spoon? Good. Now pour everything you know about bliss onto that spoon.

If you think, "I don't know anything about bliss," just use the word *bliss*. This may sound silly, I know—but it's also light and sweet and good for you, so let's do it anyway. Stir bliss into your water.

Stir. Stir. Stir. Drink it.

Raining down upon you, like divine water from the heavens...bliss.

Louise Hay, author of *You Can Heal Your Life*, writes the probable cause of ankle problems is "inflexibility and guilt. Ankles represent the ability to receive pleasure."

The remedy, according to Hay, is what she calls a new thought pattern: "I deserve to rejoice in life. I accept all the pleasure life has to offer."

Bliss is your birthright. Accept, taste, swallow it. Feel it.

11.5 Journaling

Ask yourself, "What feeling (emotion, thought, sensation) am I experiencing right now? In this moment, I feel _____."

And when you feel this way, you can choose to cultivate its opposite. Cultivating opposites is a way of attaining inner balance and bliss. It is a way of practicing non-attachment and moving beyond the pairs of opposites (praise and blame, good and bad, and many more) into more freedom.

Cultivating opposites eases us away from an "us against them" warrior mentality, which is a symptom of duality consciousness, and eases us into the powerful, peaceful inner state of unity consciousness.

Unity consciousness is blissful.

I'll say it another way: The inner state of union, in which two become one, is a state of complete pleasure, joy, and bliss.

11.6 Community

Leah Kim, Aquarius

> I have dedicated my life to yoga, both as a teacher and practitioner. I have a deep, inner strength that has enabled me to get through some unimaginably difficult times.
>
> I've experienced issues with many of my major joints, primarily due to my hyper-mobility. My right ankle always makes a popping noise when I turn it in a circle, and a couple of years ago, I sprained it quite badly.
>
> In hindsight, I now realize that that time in my life was one of great transition and fluctuation. There was probably some zodiac correlation there!
>
> I love astrology, and I check in regularly with my astrologist. I find it fascinating how there are always connections between what's written in the stars and what manifests in my life.
>
> Astrology ascribes a sense of meaning and a sense of calm.

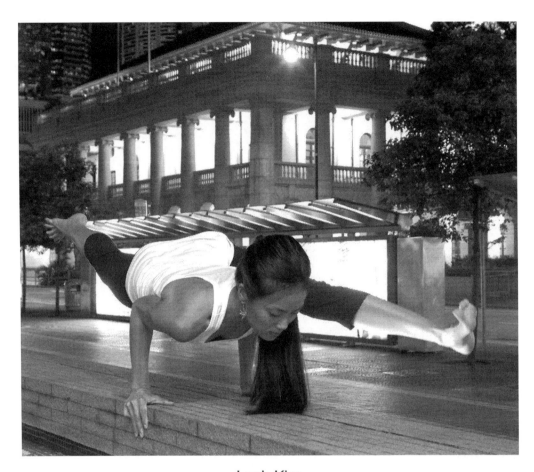

Leah Kim

11.7 Affirmation

I practice radical self-acceptance.

Don't run around the world looking for a hole to hide in. There are wild beasts in every cave. If you live with mice, the cat's claws will find you. The only real rest comes when you are alone with your Self. Live in the nowhere that you came from, even though you have an address here. That's why you see things in two ways. Everyone is half and half and both are right.
-Rumi

12 pisces: FEET

Sun in Pisces: February 19 to March 20

Welcome to Pisces Yogastrology. This chapter leads you to get grounded, explore your foundations, and dream big. Then manifest your dreams.

12.1 Element, Overview, Ruling Planet: Neptune
12.2 Traditional Body–Zodiac Correlation: Feet
12.3 Wellness: Asanas
12.4 Exploration: Neptunian Enlightenment or Escapism
12.5 Journaling: What's it like to be swept off your feet?
12.6 Community: Dani Byrne McGuire, Pisces; and Nancy Kate Williams Rau, Pisces
12.7 Affirmation: I am living my dream.

The final sign of the zodiac is a land of mystery and manifestation, illusion and disillusionment, dreams and delights.

12.1 Pisces Element, Overview, Ruling Planet

Pisces is a water sign; and the word "pisces" is the Latin word for fish. A fish symbol is used to denote Pisces—usually it is two fishes, swimming in opposite directions. A fish symbol is used to depict Christianity, too, usually seen as the outline of one fish. It's curious how often spirituality is associated with fish.

It's also curious how often spirituality is associated with feet. Ancient yogic teachings claim that feet are an especially potent spiritual center in the body.

Traits associated with Pisces include qualities of the spirit: idealism, generosity, creativity, and kindness. The Piscean influence can make a person respond to suffering with deep sympathy and tenderness, but this heightened sensitivity also can indicate an escapist tendency.

Pisces love art, music, poetry, or religion, and they also may love spirits, such as alcohol or drugs.

The Piscean influence invites a curious mixture of impracticality, extreme imagination, and spirituality.

Ruling planet: Neptune

Perhaps best known as the Lord of the Sea—also called the planet of mystery, illusion, and disillusion—glamorous and spiritual Neptune represents our longing (and our attempts) to escape the mundane world.

This planet's influence beckons us from some far-away land, drawing us toward an idealized realm where our inner dreamer can come out and play.

Neptune's influence invites you to indulge in fantasy and enjoy a dream world of vast proportions. Sail off into the sunset; drown in sublime ecstasy.

Let yourself be wild and dream big. Gloria Steinem said, "Dreaming, after all, is part of planning." And then get grounded and become solid in your foundation again; manifest those big dreams. Yoga leads the way.

12.2 Traditional Body–Zodiac Correlation

Pisces: Feet

Also: Immune system, lymphatic system, and the pineal gland

12.3 Wellness: Asanas

Grounded is a term we hear a lot these days. It's usually used to talk about the qualities of stability and firmness.

Getting, being, or staying grounded are choices we can make. We can choose to be grounded, or not, depending on what serves us at the time.

Groundedness is available to you and to me at any moment, as long as we know how to inhabit our bodies, as yoga teaches us to do. The feeling of being grounded can come as a welcome relief, like aahhhh...I've come home.

Getting grounded is a good thing, right? When I was a kid, getting grounded meant discipline. When my sisters and I were naughty, we got grounded and had to go inside (the house) and stay there for a while.

It's interesting to reconsider what it means to get grounded in yoga.

All yoga is good. For Pisces, practice any asana (at any level, beginner to advanced, whatever is appropriate for you) while maintaining focus on the feet. You might try the following practices:

Matsyasana, fish pose

Tadasana, mountain pose

Ardha Bhekasana, half frog pose

Urdhva Prasarita Eka Padasana, standing split

Supta Padangusthasana, reclining big toe pose

Urdhva Mukha Svanasana, upward-facing dog pose

Adho Mukha Svanasana, downward-facing dog pose

Featured Asana: *Utthita Hasta Padangustasana,* extended hand-to-big-toe pose

In balance poses such as Utthita Hasta Padangustasana (and all standing poses, for that matter), maintaining solid grounding through the standing leg and foot helps us stay steady and serene in the pose— and that translates into steadiness and serenity in our lives.

12.4 Exploration

Think of the timeless legends that surround the sea: tales of romance, songs of seduction; forever the temptation to sail off into the sunset, swept off your feet by a wave of passion.

If you've ever landed in the Land of Seduction, Neptune's domain, you know.

It is very hard to set up camp in Neptune's domain. Nothing lasts too long. Nor does one linger long enough to grow old.

That is the beauty of Neptune.

And yet, from time to time, the truth is that we need Neptune's inspiration. We need dreaminess, freshness, and newness, unrestrained opening to unexplored realms. Neptune evokes these processes, which are necessary in our lives.

More than we may ever know, we refresh ourselves with these fantasies.

Just be aware: Inevitably, eventually, we must emerge from these fairytale seascapes to meander back home, settling once again in the earthbound domain.

12.5 Journaling

Ask yourself, "What is it like to be swept off my feet?"

Talk about being swept off your feet! And then, getting back on your feet. Body imagery really works to make a point.

But before someone puts his foot in his mouth, let's go a-head (alright, you get the picture) and note what it means to you when you hear these words:

- Stand on your own two feet.
- Be swept off your feet.
- Get back on your feet.

And remember, there is no such thing as defeat; don't listen to any talk of defeat. Unless, of course, it's some cutie pie who wants to kiss detoes and massage defeet.

12.6 Community

Dani Byrne McGuire, Pisces

> Besides being like every other Pisces who loves to have their feet rubbed, for me being a Pisces is about staying grounded in the world while experiencing my creative essence and living a devotional life.

Naturally mystical in nature, it is easy for us Pisces to feel disconnected and ungrounded. My favorite thing to do in the warmer months is to walk through the grass each morning and feel connected to the earth. It resets me for the day, as I set the intention to experience gratitude and feel my feet firmly planted on the ground.

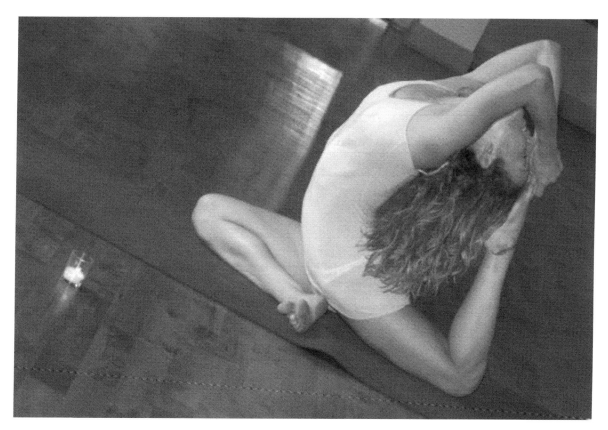

Dani Byrne McGuire

Nancy Kate Williams Rau, Pisces

Always be willing to begin again.

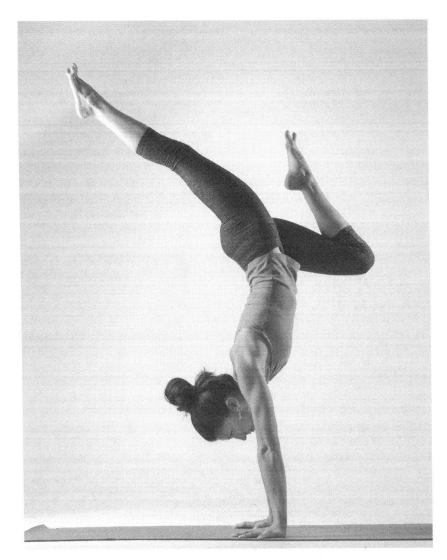

Nancy Kate Williams Rau

12.7 Affirmation

I am living my dream.

This is love: to fly toward a secret sky,
to cause a hundred veils to fall each moment.
First, to let go of life. In the end, to take a step without feet.
-Rumi

NAMASTÉ

The Four Elements: Fire, Earth, Air, and Water

Fire Element: Spirit

Yogastrology for the Fire Signs
Chapter One, Aries
Chapter Five, Leo
Chapter Nine, Sagittarius

By Molly Hall | Used by permission of the author

> Fire signs act as catalysts. The spark of fire is contagious, and we need fire to feel passionate about what we're doing.

Fire helps us burn through self-doubt and karma and it's the conduit for acting on what makes us feel alive. When there's too much fire, you are in danger of burning out.

Earth Element: Body

Yogastrology for the Earth Signs
Chapter Two, Taurus
Chapter Six, Virgo
Chapter Ten, Capricorn

Earth signs are practical. When we're balanced in earth, we feel competent and able to progress toward tangible goals.

Earth helps us be embodied–in our bodies–to revel in sensuality, luxuries, and natural pleasures. When there's too much earth, you feel heavy or lethargic.

Air Element: Intellect

Yogastrology for the Air Signs
Chapter Three, Gemini
Chapter Seven, Libra
Chapter Eleven, Aquarius

Air signs are mentally restless and idea-oriented, social, and emotionally detached (which can help you make good decisions).

When the air is moving, it makes for lively sociability and keeps you curious and always learning. When there's too much air, it's hard to feel grounded and in your body.

Water Element: Emotion

Yogastrology for the Water Signs
Chapter Four, Cancer
Chapter Eight, Scorpio
Chapter Twelve, Pisces

Water signs are attuned with intimacy, nurturance, and compassion: water purifies and cleanses. It is used to baptize, sanctify, and bless as well as to seek out the succulent and the refreshing.

Too much water and we're waterlogged, unable to see with detachment and heavy with emotional baggage. Too little water and we're dry, brittle, or despairing and feel deserted or harsh with ourselves and others.

The Four Seasons

Rejuvenate yourself with fresh seasonal practices.

Spring Equinox (March 21): Aries Yogastrology
Summer Solstice (June 22): Cancer Yogastrology

Autumnal Equinox (September 23): Libra Yogastrology
Winter Solstice (December 22): Capricorn Yogastrology

The earth is tilted on its axis, and that means the seasons are flip-flopped: in the southern hemisphere, spring/autumn are reversed and summer/winter are reversed (for example, in the southern hemisphere, spring begins in September).

Equinoxes: Spring, Autumn

Yogastrology for the Equinoxes
Chapter One, Aries
Chapter Seven, Libra

"Equinox" means equal night. On Spring Equinox and on Autumn Equinox, light equals dark. The days and nights are of equal length, in balance.

Enjoy Yogastrology for Aries and Libra.

Solstices: Summer, Winter

Yogastrology for the Solstices
Chapter Four, Cancer
Chapter Ten, Capricorn

"Solstice" means sun setting (or standing) still. This is a time to set aside routine activities and celebrate the beauty and bounty of nature.

Indulge in Yogastrology for Cancer and Capricorn.

Summer Solstice

Summer Solstice is a high-spirited time, when solar light is at its most powerful, radiant, and celebrated. There are fire dances, bonfires, and a long tradition of ritual bathing, dipping in the cleansing waters.

Celebrate water (zodiac sign Cancer is a water sign).

Winter Solstice

Winter Solstice is a sacred and rich time. The dark before the dawn can be a powerful moment of magic, drawing in what you'd like to see happen in the new year and setting intentions. The darkness itself is the spiritual cradle, a sacred time of rest before the awakening. This time of year is associated with (decorative) lights, reminders of the inner light.

Honor the earth (zodiac sign Capricorn is an earth sign).

Namasté

I hope that you've enjoyed this introduction to Yogastrology.

May it lead you to greater happiness and richer empowerment, in sync with the rhythms of nature, attuned with the four elements: the passion of fire, the generosity of earth, the freshness of mountain air, and the soothing nurturance of deep waters.

Namasté and much love,

Diane

Made in the USA
Lexington, KY
15 June 2014